30 Day POWER WEIGHT LOSS Recipes

FRANK A. KELEMEN

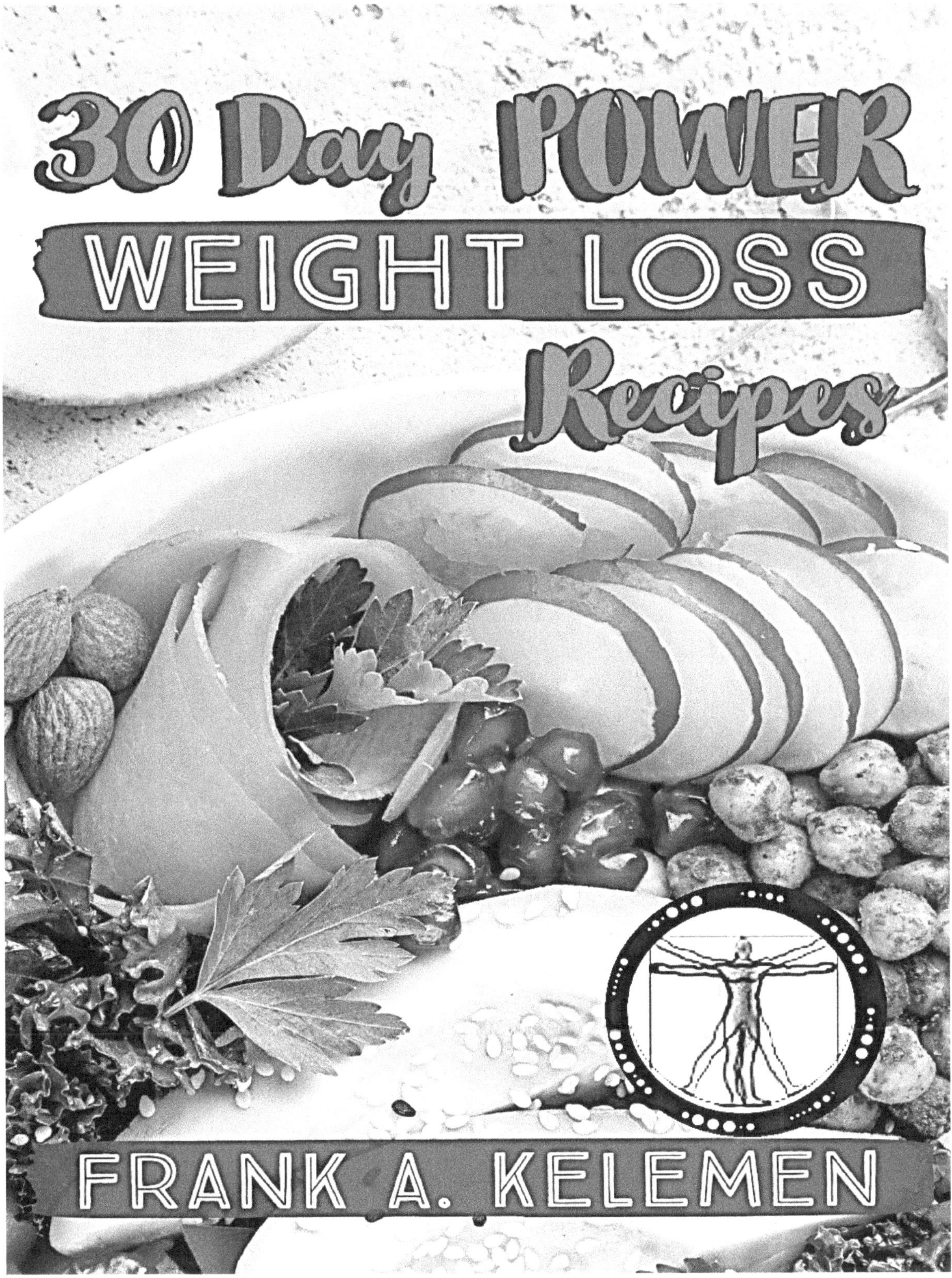

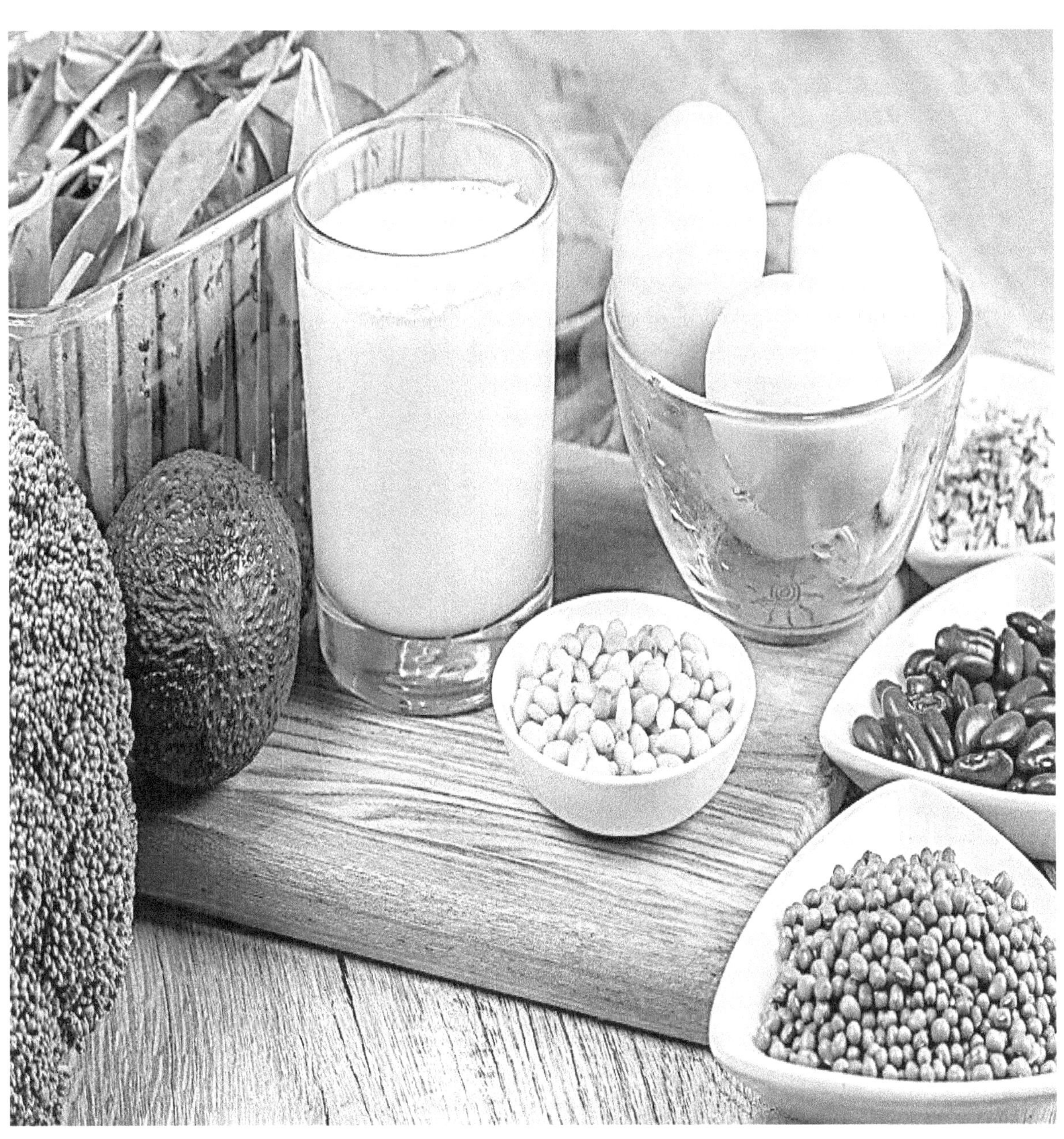

Contents

POWER Meal Weight Loss Meal Plan

Benefits

1. Balanced Nutrition:

- The meal plan provides a careful balance of macronutrients (proteins, carbohydrates, and fats) and micronutrients (vitamins and minerals).

- Proteins are essential for muscle maintenance and repair, and come from sources like chicken, fish, eggs, and legumes.

- Carbohydrates, primarily from whole grains and vegetables, provide energy and dietary fibcr.

- Healthy fats from sources like avocados, nuts, and olive oil support hormone production and nutrient absorption.

- The variety of fruits and vegetables ensures a wide spectrum of vitamins and minerals, supporting overall health and bodily functions.

2. Portion Control:

- Each meal is carefully portioned to provide adequate nutrition while supporting weight management goals.

- Consistent portion sizes help retrain the body and mind to recognize appropriate serving amounts.

- This approach prevents overeating and promotes a healthier relationship with food.

- Over time, portion control becomes more intuitive, supporting long-term healthy eating habits.

3. Weight Management:

- The balanced, calorie-controlled meals support gradual, sustainable weight loss or maintenance.

- High-fiber foods and lean proteins promote satiety, reducing overall calorie intake naturally.

- The plan's focus on whole foods helps stabilize blood sugar and insulin levels, which can aid in weight management.

- Regular meal times and balanced nutrition can boost metabolism, further supporting weight management efforts.

4. Increased Fiber Intake:

- The emphasis on whole grains, fruits, and vegetables significantly increases dietary fiber intake.

- Soluble fiber helps lower cholesterol and stabilize blood sugar levels.

- Insoluble fiber promotes regular bowel movements and digestive health.

- High-fiber diets are associated with reduced risk of heart disease, stroke, and certain types of cancer.

- Fiber also promotes feelings of fullness, which can aid in weight management.

5. Heart Health:

- The inclusion of fatty fish like salmon provides omega-3 fatty acids, which have anti-inflammatory properties and can reduce the risk of heart disease.

- Nuts, seeds, and olive oil offer heart-healthy monounsaturated and polyunsaturated fats.

- The plan limits saturated fats and eliminates trans fats, both of which are associated with increased heart disease risk.

- High fiber intake from whole grains and vegetables can help lower cholesterol levels.

- The emphasis on whole foods naturally reduces sodium intake, supporting healthy blood pressure.

6. Blood Sugar Management:

- The balance of complex carbohydrates, lean proteins, and healthy fats in each meal helps prevent rapid spikes in blood sugar.

- Consistent meal timing helps regulate insulin production and sensitivity.

- High-fiber foods slow down the absorption of sugars, leading to more stable blood glucose levels.

- This approach can be particularly beneficial for individuals with or at risk of type 2 diabetes.

- Over time, stable blood sugar can reduce cravings and support overall metabolic health.

7. Increased Vegetable and Fruit Consumption:

   - The plan incorporates a wide variety of colorful fruits and vegetables in every meal.

   - Different colors indicate various phytonutrients and antioxidants, each offering unique health benefits.

   - Increased vegetable intake is associated with reduced risk of chronic diseases, including certain cancers.

   - The high water and fiber content of fruits and vegetables supports hydration and digestive health.

   - Vitamins and minerals from produce support immune function, skin health, and overall vitality.

8. Hydration:

   - While not explicitly stated in each meal, the plan encourages increased water intake throughout the day.

   - Proper hydration supports all bodily functions, including metabolism and cognitive performance.

   - Water can help with appetite control, as thirst is often mistaken for hunger.

   - Adequate hydration supports skin health, joint lubrication, and temperature regulation.

   - Drinking water instead of high-calorie beverages can significantly reduce overall calorie intake.

9. Meal Planning and Preparation Skills:

   - Following this plan helps develop crucial meal planning skills, promoting long-term healthy eating habits.

   - Learning to prepare balanced meals enhances cooking skills and nutritional knowledge.

   - Meal planning reduces reliance on convenience foods and impulsive eating decisions.

   - These skills can lead to time and cost savings in the long run.

- The ability to plan and prepare healthy meals is a valuable life skill that can benefit the entire household.

10. Variety and Flexibility:

- The plan offers a wide range of recipes and meal ideas to prevent dietary boredom.

- Nutritional diversity ensures a broad spectrum of nutrients and phytochemicals.

- The variety of foods and preparation methods can expand culinary horizons and food preferences.

- The plan can be adapted to different dietary needs or preferences with minor modifications.

- Flexibility in the plan allows for occasional treats or dining out without derailing overall progress.

11. Reduced Processed Food Intake:

- The focus on whole foods naturally reduces consumption of processed items high in unhealthy fats, added sugars, and sodium.

- Fewer processed foods means lower intake of artificial additives and preservatives.

- Whole foods are generally more nutrient-dense and satiating than their processed counterparts.

- Reducing processed food intake can lead to improved energy levels and overall health.

- This approach supports a more natural and less industrialized way of eating.

12. Improved Energy Levels:

- The balanced nutrition provided by the meal plan leads to more stable blood sugar levels, preventing energy crashes.

- Adequate protein intake supports muscle health and can improve physical performance.

- Complex carbohydrates provide sustained energy throughout the day.

- Increased intake of vitamins and minerals supports cellular energy production.

- Proper hydration, encouraged by the plan, is crucial for maintaining energy levels.

13. Better Sleep:

- A balanced diet with proper nutrition can contribute to improved sleep quality.

- Avoiding large meals close to bedtime can prevent discomfort and acid reflux that might disrupt sleep.

- The tryptophan found in some of the plan's protein sources can promote better sleep.

- Reduced intake of processed foods and added sugars may lead to more restful sleep.

- Consistent meal times help regulate the body's internal clock, which can improve sleep patterns.

14. Sustainable Eating Habits:

- The plan introduces a sustainable approach to healthy eating that can be maintained long-term.

- It focuses on lifestyle changes rather than restrictive, short-term dieting.

- The variety and flexibility of the plan make it easier to adhere to over time.

- Learning to prepare balanced meals supports long-term healthy eating habits.

- The plan can be adjusted over time to meet changing nutritional needs or goals.

15. Cost-Effective:

- Meal planning and preparing foods at home is generally more cost-effective than eating out or buying pre-prepared meals.

- Buying whole foods in bulk can lead to significant savings.

- Reduced food waste through planned meals and proper portioning saves money.

- Investing in health through proper nutrition can lead to long-term healthcare cost savings.

- The skills learned through this plan can continue to provide financial benefits well beyond the 30 days.

Remember, while this meal plan offers many benefits, individual results may vary based on factors such as starting health status, adherence to the plan, and lifestyle factors. It's always recommended to consult with a healthcare professional or registered dietitian before starting any new diet plan, especially for individuals with specific health concerns or dietary requirements.

Weight Loss on the POWER Diet

The rate of weight loss can vary from person to person, but here are typical weight loss data for an average person:

Week 1: 2-4 lbs (0.9-1.8 kg)

Week 2: 1-2 lbs (0.45-0.9 kg)

Week 3: 1-2 lbs (0.45-0.9 kg)

Week 4: 1-2 lbs (0.45-0.9 kg)

Total expected weight loss over 30 days: 5-10 lbs (2.3-4.5 kg).

These numbers are based on general expectations for healthy weight loss. It's important to note that individual results may vary depending on factors such as starting weight, adherence to the diet, exercise intensity, and individual metabolism.

Consistency, patience, and regular monitoring of progress are crucial for sustainable weight loss on the keto diet. It's also essential to consult with a healthcare professional, especially if you have any underlying medical conditions, to ensure the keto diet is appropriate and safe for you.

30 Day POWER Meal Plan

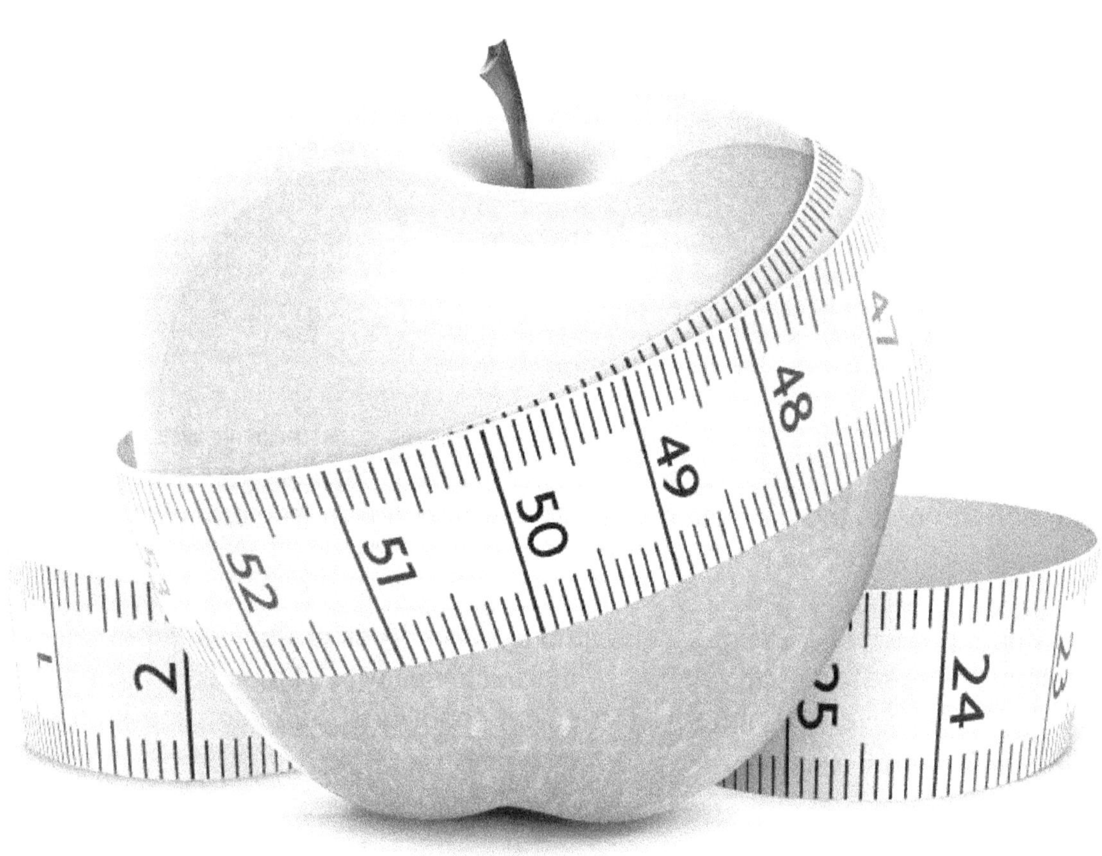

Day 1

Breakfast: Oatmeal with berries and almonds

Macronutrients: 350 calories, 12g protein, 50g carbs, 14g fat

Recipe:

1. In a pot, combine 1/2 cup rolled oats with 1 cup water or milk.

2. Bring to a boil, then reduce heat and simmer for 5 minutes, stirring occasionally.

3. Remove from heat and let stand for 2 minutes.

4. Transfer to a bowl and top with 1/2 cup mixed berries (strawberries, blueberries, raspberries) and 1 tbsp sliced almonds.

5. Optional: Add a drizzle of honey for sweetness.

Lunch: Grilled chicken salad

Macronutrients: 400 calories, 35g protein, 20g carbs, 22g fat

Recipe:

1. Season 4 oz chicken breast with salt, pepper, and Italian herbs.

2. Grill the chicken for 6-7 minutes per side until internal temperature reaches 165°F (74°C).

3. While chicken is cooking, prepare the salad: mix 2 cups mixed greens, 1/2 cup sliced cucumber, 1/2 cup cherry tomatoes, and 1/4 sliced red onion.

4. For the dressing, whisk together 1 tbsp olive oil, 1 tbsp balsamic vinegar, 1 tsp Dijon mustard, and a pinch of salt and pepper.

5. Slice the grilled chicken and place on top of the salad.

6. Drizzle with the prepared dressing.

Dinner: Baked salmon with roasted vegetables

Macronutrients: 450 calories, 30g protein, 25g carbs, 28g fat

Recipe:

1. Preheat oven to 400°F (200°C).

2. Place a 4 oz salmon fillet on a baking sheet lined with parchment paper.

3. Season salmon with salt, pepper, and dried herbs (like dill or thyme). Place lemon slices on top.

4. On the same baking sheet, add 1 cup mixed vegetables (broccoli florets, sliced carrots, zucchini chunks). Toss with 1 tbsp olive oil, salt, and pepper.

5. Bake for 12-15 minutes until salmon is cooked through and vegetables are tender.

Day 2

Breakfast Greek yogurt parfait

Macronutrients: 400 calories, 25g protein, 50g carbs, 14g fat

Recipe:

1. In a glass or bowl, layer 1 cup plain Greek yogurt with 1/2 cup low-fat granola.

2. Add 1/2 cup mixed fruit (e.g., sliced strawberries, blueberries, and peaches).

3. Optional: Drizzle with 1 tsp honey for added sweetness.

Lunch: Turkey and avocado wrap

Macronutrients: 380 calories, 25g protein, 35g carbs, 18g fat

Recipe:

1. Lay out a whole grain wrap on a clean surface.

2. Spread 1/4 mashed avocado on the wrap.

3. Layer 3 oz sliced turkey breast, 2 slices of tomato, and a handful of lettuce leaves.

4. Optionally, add a spread of 1 tsp Dijon mustard for extra flavor.

5. Roll the wrap tightly, tucking in the sides as you go.

6. Cut in half diagonally and serve.

Dinner: Vegetarian chili

Macronutrients: 420 calories, 18g protein, 65g carbs, 12g fat

Recipe:

1. In a large pot, heat 1 tbsp olive oil over medium heat.

2. Sauté 1/2 diced onion and 1 minced garlic clove until softened.

3. Add 1 diced bell pepper and cook for another 2 minutes.

4. Stir in 1 can (15 oz) diced tomatoes, 1 can (15 oz) mixed beans (drained and rinsed), 1 cup vegetable broth, 1 tbsp chili powder, 1 tsp cumin, and salt to taste.

5. Simmer for 20-25 minutes, stirring occasionally.

6. Serve with a small side salad of mixed greens and a light vinaigrette.

Day 3

Breakfast: Vegetable omelet

Macronutrients: 350 calories, 25g protein, 20g carbs, 22g fat

Recipe:

1. Whisk 2 eggs with a splash of milk, salt, and pepper.

2. Heat a non-stick pan over medium heat and add 1 tsp olive oil.

3. Sauté 1/4 cup chopped spinach and 1/4 cup sliced mushrooms until softened.

4. Pour the egg mixture over the vegetables and cook until edges are set.

5. Sprinkle 1 tbsp shredded cheese over half the omelet, fold, and cook until cheese melts.

6. Serve with 1 slice whole grain toast.

Lunch: Quinoa bowl

Macronutrients: 400 calories, 15g protein, 60g carbs, 16g fat

Recipe:

1. Cook 1/2 cup quinoa according to package instructions.

2. Grill or roast 1 cup mixed vegetables (zucchini, bell peppers, eggplant).

3. Heat 3 oz canned chickpeas (drained and rinsed) in a pan with a pinch of cumin and paprika.

4. For tahini dressing, mix 1 tbsp tahini with 1 tbsp lemon juice and 1 tbsp water.

5. Assemble the bowl: quinoa, grilled vegetables, chickpeas, and drizzle with tahini dressing.

Dinner: Grilled lean steak with sweet potato

Macronutrients: 450 calories, 35g protein, 40g carbs, 18g fat

Recipe:

1. Season a 4 oz lean steak with salt and pepper.

2. Grill for 3-4 minutes each side for medium-rare, or to desired doneness.

3. Pierce a small sweet potato with a fork and microwave for 5-7 minutes until soft.

4. Steam 1 cup green beans for 3-4 minutes until crisp-tender.

5. Serve steak with sweet potato and green beans.

Day 4

Breakfast: Whole grain toast with avocado and poached egg

Macronutrients: 380 calories, 18g protein, 30g carbs, 24g fat

Recipe:

- 1 slice whole grain bread, toasted

- 1/4 avocado, mashed

- 1 poached egg

- Salt and pepper to taste

Spread mashed avocado on toast, top with poached egg, season with salt and pepper.

Lunch: Tuna salad lettuce wraps

Macronutrients: 350 calories, 30g protein, 15g carbs, 20g fat

Recipe:

- 1 can (5 oz) tuna in water, drained

- 1 tbsp Greek yogurt

- 1 tbsp mayo

- 1/4 cup diced celery

- 1 tbsp diced red onion

- 1 tsp lemon juice

- Salt and pepper to taste

- 4 large lettuce leaves

Mix all ingredients except lettuce. Divide mixture among lettuce leaves.

Dinner: Stir-fry tofu with mixed vegetables

Macronutrients: 400 calories, 20g protein, 45g carbs, 20g fat

Recipe:

- 7 oz firm tofu, cubed

- 2 cups mixed vegetables (bell peppers, broccoli, carrots)

- 1 tbsp olive oil

- 1 tbsp low-sodium soy sauce

- 1 tsp sesame oil

- 1 clove garlic, minced

- 1/2 tsp ginger, grated

Heat oils in a pan, stir-fry tofu until golden. Add vegetables, garlic, and ginger. Cook until tender-crisp. Add soy sauce and toss to combine.

Day 5

Breakfast: Smoothie bowl (banana, berries, spinach, Greek yogurt, almond milk)

Macronutrients: 350 calories, 20g protein, 55g carbs, 10g fat

Recipe:

- 1 ripe banana

- 1/2 cup mixed berries

- 1 cup spinach

- 1/2 cup Greek yogurt

- 1/4 cup unsweetened almond milk

- Optional toppings: chia seeds, sliced almonds

Blend all ingredients except toppings until smooth. Pour into a bowl and add toppings if desired.

Lunch: Lentil soup with whole grain roll

Macronutrients: 380 calories, 18g protein, 60g carbs, 8g fat

Recipe:

- 1/2 cup dry lentils

- 2 cups vegetable broth

- 1/4 cup diced onion

- 1/4 cup diced carrot

- 1/4 cup diced celery

- 1 clove garlic, minced

- 1 tsp olive oil

- 1/2 tsp cumin

- Salt and pepper to taste

- 1 small whole grain roll

Sauté vegetables in oil. Add lentils, broth, and seasonings. Simmer until lentils are tender. Serve with roll.

Dinner: Grilled chicken breast with quinoa and roasted Brussels sprouts

Macronutrients: 420 calories, 35g protein, 40g carbs, 15g fat

Recipe:

- 4 oz chicken breast

- 1/2 cup cooked quinoa

- 1 cup Brussels sprouts, halved

- 1 tbsp olive oil

- 1 tsp lemon juice

- 1 clove garlic, minced

- Salt and pepper to taste

Season chicken with garlic, salt, and pepper. Grill until cooked through. Toss Brussels sprouts with oil, salt, and pepper; roast at 400°F for 20-25 minutes. Serve chicken over quinoa with Brussels sprouts on the side.

Day 6

Breakfast: Protein pancakes

Macronutrients: 380 calories, 25g protein, 45g carbs, 14g fat

Recipe:

1. In a bowl, mix 1/2 cup rolled oats, 2 egg whites, 1/2 mashed banana, 1/4 cup cottage cheese, 1 tsp baking powder, and a pinch of cinnamon.

2. Heat a non-stick pan over medium heat and lightly coat with cooking spray.

3. Pour batter to make 3-4 small pancakes. Cook for 2-3 minutes each side until golden brown.

4. Top with 1/4 cup mixed berries and 1 tbsp sugar-free maple syrup.

Lunch: Grilled vegetable and hummus wrap

Macronutrients: 400 calories, 15g protein, 50g carbs, 20g fat

Recipe:

1. Grill or roast 1 cup mixed vegetables (zucchini, bell peppers, eggplant) with 1 tsp olive oil and seasoning.

2. Warm a whole wheat wrap in a dry pan.

3. Spread 2 tbsp hummus on the wrap.

4. Add grilled vegetables and 1/4 cup baby spinach leaves.

5. Roll tightly and cut in half diagonally.

Dinner: Baked cod with roasted vegetables

Macronutrients: 420 calories, 35g protein, 30g carbs, 18g fat

Recipe:

1. Preheat oven to 400°F (200°C).

2. Season a 5 oz cod fillet with salt, pepper, and lemon juice.

3. On a baking sheet, toss 1.5 cups mixed vegetables (broccoli, carrots, Brussels sprouts) with 1 tbsp olive oil, salt, and pepper.

4. Place cod on the same baking sheet.

5. Bake for 15-18 minutes until cod is flaky and vegetables are tender.

Day 7

Breakfast: Veggie scramble

Macronutrients: 350 calories, 22g protein, 25g carbs, 20g fat

Recipe:

1. In a bowl, whisk 2 whole eggs and 1 egg white with salt and pepper.

2. Heat 1 tsp olive oil in a non-stick pan over medium heat.

3. Sauté 1/4 cup each of diced bell peppers, onions, and spinach until softened.

4. Pour the egg mixture over the vegetables and stir gently until eggs are set.

5. Serve with 1 slice whole grain toast and 1/4 sliced avocado.

Lunch: Chicken and quinoa bowl

Macronutrients: 420 calories, 35g protein, 45g carbs, 14g fat

Recipe:

1. Cook 1/2 cup quinoa according to package instructions.

2. Grill 4 oz chicken breast seasoned with herbs and spices.

3. Steam 1 cup mixed vegetables (broccoli, carrots, snap peas).

4. In a bowl, combine quinoa, sliced grilled chicken, and steamed vegetables.

5. Drizzle with 1 tbsp lemon-tahini dressing (mix 1 tbsp tahini, 1 tsp lemon juice, 1 tsp water).

Dinner: Vegetarian lentil loaf

Macronutrients: 400 calories, 20g protein, 60g carbs, 12g fat

Recipe:

1. Preheat oven to 375°F (190°C).

2. In a bowl, mix 1 cup cooked lentils, 1/2 cup cooked quinoa, 1/4 cup breadcrumbs, 1 beaten egg, 1/4 cup diced onion, 1 minced garlic clove, 1 tbsp tomato paste, and seasonings.

3. Press mixture into a loaf pan lined with parchment paper.

4. Bake for 30-35 minutes until firm and golden on top.

5. Serve with a side salad of mixed greens and balsamic vinaigrette.

Day 8

Breakfast: Chia seed pudding

Macronutrients: 340 calories, 14g protein, 45g carbs, 16g fat

Recipe:

1. In a jar, mix 3 tbsp chia seeds with 1 cup unsweetened almond milk and 1 tsp vanilla extract.

2. Refrigerate overnight or for at least 4 hours.

3. In the morning, stir the pudding and add 1/2 cup mixed berries and 1 tbsp sliced almonds.

4. Optional: Drizzle with 1 tsp honey for added sweetness.

Lunch: Mediterranean salad with feta

Macronutrients: 380 calories, 15g protein, 30g carbs, 25g fat

Recipe:

1. In a large bowl, combine 2 cups mixed greens, 1/2 cup diced cucumber, 1/4 cup halved cherry tomatoes, 1/4 cup diced bell pepper, 2 tbsp sliced red onion, and 10 kalamata olives.

2. Add 1/4 cup crumbled feta cheese and 2 tbsp chickpeas.

3. Dress with 1 tbsp olive oil and 1 tsp lemon juice, mixed with dried oregano, salt, and pepper.

4. Toss all ingredients together and serve.

Dinner: Shrimp stir-fry

Macronutrients: 400 calories, 30g protein, 40g carbs, 15g fat

Recipe:

1. In a wok or large pan, heat 1 tbsp vegetable oil over medium-high heat.

2. Add 4 oz peeled and deveined shrimp, cook for 2-3 minutes until pink.

3. Remove shrimp and set aside.

4. In the same pan, stir-fry 1.5 cups mixed vegetables (bell peppers, broccoli, snap peas, carrots) for 3-4 minutes.

5. Add 1 minced garlic clove and 1 tsp grated ginger, cook for 30 seconds.

6. Return shrimp to the pan, add 1 tbsp low-sodium soy sauce and 1 tsp sesame oil.

7. Serve over 1/2 cup cooked brown rice.

Day 9

Breakfast: Whole grain cereal with milk and fruit

Macronutrients: 360 calories, 15g protein, 60g carbs, 8g fat

Recipe:

1. In a bowl, pour 1 cup whole grain cereal (like bran flakes or shredded wheat).

2. Add 1 cup low-fat milk or unsweetened plant-based milk.

3. Top with 1/2 cup mixed berries (strawberries, blueberries, raspberries).

4. Optional: Add 1 tbsp chopped nuts for extra protein and healthy fats.

Lunch: Black bean burrito bowl

Macronutrients: 420 calories, 18g protein, 65g carbs, 14g fat

Recipe:

1. Cook 1/2 cup brown rice according to package instructions.

2. In a pan, heat 1/2 cup canned black beans (drained and rinsed) with 1/4 tsp cumin and 1/4 tsp chili powder.

3. Dice 1/4 avocado and 1/4 cup tomatoes.

4. Assemble the bowl: rice, black beans, diced avocado, tomatoes, 2 tbsp corn, and 1/4 cup shredded lettuce.

5. Top with 2 tbsp salsa and 1 tbsp plain Greek yogurt as a sour cream substitute.

Dinner: Lean beef stew

Macronutrients: 450 calories, 35g protein, 40g carbs, 18g fat

Recipe:

1. In a pot, brown 4 oz lean beef cubes in 1 tsp olive oil.

2. Add 1/2 diced onion and 1 minced garlic clove, cook until softened.

3. Add 1 cup beef broth, 1/2 cup diced tomatoes, 1 diced carrot, 1 diced potato, and 1/2 cup green beans.

4. Season with 1 bay leaf, 1/2 tsp thyme, salt, and pepper.

5. Simmer for 1-1.5 hours until beef is tender and vegetables are cooked.

6. Thicken with 1 tsp cornstarch mixed with water if desired.

Day 10

Breakfast: Greek yogurt with granola

Macronutrients: 380 calories, 25g protein, 45g carbs, 12g fat

Recipe:

1. In a bowl, add 1 cup plain Greek yogurt.

2. Top with 1/4 cup low-fat granola.

3. Add 1/2 sliced banana and 1/4 cup mixed berries.

4. Drizzle with 1 tsp honey if desired.

Lunch: Turkey and avocado sandwich

Macronutrients: 400 calories, 25g protein, 35g carbs, 20g fat

Recipe:

1. Toast 2 slices of whole grain bread.

2. Spread 1/4 mashed avocado on one slice of bread.

3. Layer 3 oz sliced turkey breast, 1 slice tomato, and a handful of lettuce leaves.

4. Spread 1 tsp mustard on the other slice of bread and assemble the sandwich.

5. Serve with a small side of baby carrots or cucumber slices.

Dinner: Grilled portobello mushroom caps

Macronutrients: 350 calories, 15g protein, 40g carbs, 18g fat

Recipe:

1. Clean and remove stems from 2 large portobello mushroom caps.

2. Brush mushrooms with 1 tsp olive oil and season with garlic powder, salt, and pepper.

3. Grill for 4-5 minutes per side until tender.

4. Meanwhile, cook 1/2 cup quinoa according to package instructions.

5. In a small bowl, mix 2 tbsp crumbled feta cheese with 1 tbsp chopped fresh basil.

6. Serve grilled mushrooms over quinoa, topped with the feta mixture.

7. Serve with a side of grilled or steamed zucchini.

Day 11

Breakfast: Breakfast burrito

Macronutrients: 400 calories, 25g protein, 40g carbs, 18g fat

Recipe:

1. Scramble 1 whole egg and 2 egg whites with salt and pepper.

2. In a separate pan, sauté 1/4 cup diced bell peppers and 2 tbsp diced onions.

3. Warm a whole wheat tortilla.

4. Fill tortilla with scrambled eggs, sautéed vegetables, 2 tbsp black beans, and 2 tbsp shredded low-fat cheese.

5. Roll up tightly and serve with 2 tbsp salsa on the side.

Lunch: Turkey chili

Macronutrients: 380 calories, 30g protein, 45g carbs, 10g fat

Recipe:

1. In a pot, brown 4 oz ground turkey breast.

2. Add 1/4 cup diced onions and 1 minced garlic clove, cook until softened.

3. Stir in 1/2 cup canned diced tomatoes, 1/4 cup kidney beans, 1/4 cup corn, and 1/2 cup low-sodium chicken broth.

4. Season with 1 tsp chili powder, 1/2 tsp cumin, salt, and pepper.

5. Simmer for 20-25 minutes until flavors meld.

6. Serve topped with 1 tbsp plain Greek yogurt and chopped cilantro.

Dinner: Baked chicken parmesan

Macronutrients: 450 calories, 40g protein, 30g carbs, 20g fat

Recipe:

1. Preheat oven to 400°F (200°C).

2. Dip a 4 oz chicken breast in 1 beaten egg white, then coat with a mixture of 2 tbsp whole wheat breadcrumbs and 1 tbsp grated parmesan cheese.

3. Place on a baking sheet and bake for 20-25 minutes until cooked through.

4. Top with 2 tbsp marinara sauce and 1 oz low-fat mozzarella cheese.

5. Broil for 2-3 minutes until cheese is melted and bubbly.

6. Serve with 1 cup steamed broccoli and 1/2 cup whole wheat pasta.

Day 12

Breakfast: Cottage cheese with fruit

Macronutrients: 320 calories, 25g protein, 40g carbs, 8g fat

Recipe:

1. In a bowl, add 1 cup low-fat cottage cheese.

2. Top with 1/2 cup mixed fresh fruit (e.g., sliced peaches, strawberries, and blueberries).

3. Sprinkle with 1 tbsp chopped walnuts.

4. Optional: Drizzle with 1 tsp honey for added sweetness.

Lunch: Spinach and strawberry salad

Macronutrients: 380 calories, 20g protein, 35g carbs, 22g fat

Recipe:

1. In a large bowl, combine 3 cups baby spinach leaves with 1 cup sliced strawberries.

2. Add 1/4 cup crumbled feta cheese and 2 tbsp sliced almonds.

3. For the dressing, whisk together 1 tbsp olive oil, 1 tbsp balsamic vinegar, 1 tsp Dijon mustard, and 1 tsp honey.

4. Toss the salad with the dressing just before serving.

5. Serve with 1 small whole grain roll on the side.

Dinner. Salmon with asparagus

Macronutrients: 420 calories, 35g protein, 25g carbs, 22g fat

Recipe:

1. Preheat oven to 400°F (200°C).

2. Place a 5 oz salmon fillet on a baking sheet lined with parchment paper.

3. Season salmon with salt, pepper, and lemon zest.

4. Arrange 1 cup asparagus spears around the salmon. Drizzle with 1 tsp olive oil and season.

5. Bake for 12-15 minutes until salmon is cooked through and asparagus is tender.

6. Serve with 1/2 cup cooked quinoa and a lemon wedge.

Day 13

Breakfast: Overnight oats

Macronutrients: 380 calories, 18g protein, 55g carbs, 12g fat

Recipe:

1. In a jar, combine 1/2 cup rolled oats, 1/2 cup low-fat milk or unsweetened almond milk, 1/4 cup plain Greek yogurt, and 1 tsp chia seeds.

2. Add 1/2 mashed banana and 1/4 tsp vanilla extract.

3. Stir well, cover, and refrigerate overnight.

4. In the morning, top with 1/4 cup mixed berries and 1 tbsp chopped nuts.

Lunch: Vegetable soup with whole grain crackers

Macronutrients: 350 calories, 15g protein, 50g carbs, 12g fat

Recipe:

1. In a pot, sauté 1/4 cup each of diced onions, carrots, and celery in 1 tsp olive oil.

2. Add 2 cups low-sodium vegetable broth, 1/2 cup diced tomatoes, 1/4 cup green beans, and 1/4 cup diced zucchini.

3. Season with 1 bay leaf, 1/4 tsp thyme, salt, and pepper.

4. Simmer for 20 minutes until vegetables are tender.

5. Serve with 6-8 whole grain crackers and 1 oz low-fat cheese on the side.

Dinner: Turkey meatballs with zucchini noodles

Macronutrients: 420 calories, 35g protein, 30g carbs, 20g fat

Recipe:

1. Mix 4 oz ground turkey with 2 tbsp whole wheat breadcrumbs, 1 minced garlic clove, 1 tbsp grated Parmesan, and Italian herbs.

2. Form into small meatballs and bake at 375°F (190°C) for 15-20 minutes until cooked through.

3. Spiralize 1 medium zucchini into noodles.

4. In a pan, sauté zucchini noodles in 1 tsp olive oil for 2-3 minutes until slightly softened.

5. Heat 1/2 cup marinara sauce and toss with zucchini noodles and meatballs.

6. Garnish with fresh basil and 1 tbsp grated Parmesan cheese.

Day 14

Breakfast: Egg white frittata

Macronutrients: 300 calories, 25g protein, 20g carbs, 15g fat

Recipe:

1. Preheat oven to 375°F (190°C).

2. In a bowl, whisk 4 egg whites with salt and pepper.

3. In an oven-safe skillet, sauté 1/4 cup each of diced bell peppers, spinach, and mushrooms in 1 tsp olive oil.

4. Pour egg whites over vegetables and cook for 2 minutes on the stovetop.

5. Transfer skillet to oven and bake for 10-12 minutes until set.

6. Serve with 1 slice whole grain toast and 1/4 sliced avocado.

Lunch: Tuna Nicoise salad

Macronutrients: 400 calories, 30g protein, 35g carbs, 18g fat

Recipe:

1. Boil 1 small potato and 1/4 cup green beans until tender. Cool and cut into pieces.

2. In a bowl, combine 2 cups mixed greens, cooked potato and green beans, 1/4 cup halved cherry tomatoes, and 5 sliced olives.

3. Add 3 oz canned tuna (drained) and 1 hard-boiled egg, quartered.

4. Dress with a mixture of 1 tbsp olive oil, 1 tsp Dijon mustard, and 1 tsp red wine vinegar.

5. Toss gently and serve.

Dinner: Tofu and vegetable curry

Macronutrients: 420 calories, 20g protein, 50g carbs, 18g fat

Recipe:

1. Press and cube 4 oz firm tofu.

2. In a pan, sauté 1/4 cup diced onion and 1 minced garlic clove in 1 tsp coconut oil.

3. Add 1 tbsp curry powder and cook for 30 seconds.

4. Add 1/2 cup coconut milk, 1/4 cup vegetable broth, and 1 cup mixed vegetables (cauliflower, carrots, peas).

5. Simmer for 10 minutes, then add tofu and cook for another 5 minutes.

6. Serve over 1/2 cup cooked brown rice and garnish with fresh cilantro.

Day 15

Breakfast: Whole grain waffles with nut butter

Macronutrients: 400 calories, 18g protein, 45g carbs, 20g fat

Recipe:

1. Toast 2 whole grain frozen waffles according to package instructions.

2. Spread 1 tbsp almond or peanut butter on each waffle.

3. Top with 1/2 sliced banana and a sprinkle of cinnamon.

4. Drizzle with 1 tsp honey if desired.

Lunch: Chickpea salad

Macronutrients: 380 calories, 15g protein, 50g carbs, 18g fat

Recipe:

1. In a bowl, combine 1/2 cup canned chickpeas (drained and rinsed) with 1 cup mixed salad greens.

2. Add 1/4 cup diced cucumber, 1/4 cup cherry tomatoes, and 2 tbsp diced red onion.

3. Crumble 1 oz feta cheese over the salad.

4. For dressing, mix 1 tbsp olive oil, 1 tsp lemon juice, 1/4 tsp dried oregano, salt, and pepper.

5. Toss the salad with the dressing and serve.

Dinner: Baked chicken parmesan

Macronutrients: 450 calories, 40g protein, 30g carbs, 20g fat

Recipe:

1. Preheat oven to 400°F (200°C).

2. Dip a 4 oz chicken breast in 1 beaten egg white, then coat with a mixture of 2 tbsp whole wheat breadcrumbs and 1 tbsp grated parmesan cheese.

3. Place on a baking sheet and bake for 20-25 minutes until cooked through.

4. Top with 2 tbsp marinara sauce and 1 oz low-fat mozzarella cheese.

5. Broil for 2-3 minutes until cheese is melted and bubbly.

6. Serve with 1 cup steamed broccoli and 1/2 cup whole wheat pasta.

Day 16

Breakfast: Banana oat muffins

Macronutrients: 340 calories, 12g protein, 55g carbs, 10g fat

Recipe:

1. Preheat oven to 375°F (190°C).

2. In a bowl, mash 1 ripe banana and mix with 1 beaten egg, 1/4 cup Greek yogurt, and 2 tbsp honey.

3. In another bowl, combine 1/2 cup whole wheat flour, 1/2 cup rolled oats, 1 tsp baking powder, and 1/4 tsp cinnamon.

4. Mix wet and dry ingredients until just combined.

5. Divide batter into 6 muffin cups and bake for 18-20 minutes.

6. Enjoy 2 muffins for breakfast.

Lunch: Greek salad wrap

Macronutrients: 400 calories, 20g protein, 40g carbs, 22g fat

Recipe:

1. In a bowl, mix 1/2 cup diced cucumber, 1/4 cup diced tomatoes, 2 tbsp diced red onion, and 5 sliced kalamata olives.

2. Add 2 oz crumbled feta cheese and 1 tbsp chopped fresh parsley.

3. Drizzle with 1 tsp olive oil and 1 tsp lemon juice, mix well.

4. Warm a large whole wheat tortilla and spread with 1 tbsp hummus.

5. Add the Greek salad mixture and roll up tightly.

Dinner: Lean pork tenderloin with sweet potato mash

Macronutrients: 430 calories, 35g protein, 45g carbs, 14g fat

Recipe:

1. Preheat oven to 400°F (200°C).

2. Season a 4 oz pork tenderloin with herbs, salt, and pepper.

3. Roast for 20-25 minutes until internal temperature reaches 145°F (63°C).

4. Meanwhile, peel and cube 1 medium sweet potato. Boil until tender, about 15 minutes.

5. Mash sweet potato with 1 tbsp Greek yogurt, salt, and pepper.

6. Steam 1 cup green beans.

7. Slice pork and serve with sweet potato mash and green beans.

Day 17

Breakfast: Smoked salmon on whole grain bagel

Macronutrients: 380 calories, 25g protein, 45g carbs, 14g fat

Recipe:

1. Toast 1/2 whole grain bagel.

2. Spread with 1 tbsp low-fat cream cheese.

3. Top with 2 oz smoked salmon, 2 thin slices of red onion, and 1 tsp capers.

4. Serve with a few slices of cucumber on the side.

Lunch: Lentil and vegetable soup

Macronutrients: 350 calories, 18g protein, 55g carbs, 8g fat

Recipe:

1. In a pot, sauté 1/4 cup each diced onion, carrot, and celery in 1 tsp olive oil.

2. Add 1/2 cup dried lentils, 2 cups vegetable broth, 1/2 cup diced tomatoes, and 1 cup chopped spinach.

3. Season with 1 tsp cumin, 1/2 tsp turmeric, salt, and pepper.

4. Simmer for 25-30 minutes until lentils are tender.

5. Serve with a small whole grain roll.

Dinner: Vegetarian chili

Macronutrients: 420 calories, 18g protein, 65g carbs, 12g fat

Recipe:

1. In a pot, sauté 1/4 cup diced onion and 1 minced garlic clove in 1 tsp olive oil.

2. Add 1/2 cup each of canned black beans and kidney beans (drained and rinsed), 1/2 cup diced tomatoes, 1/4 cup corn, and 1/2 cup vegetable broth.

3. Season with 1 tbsp chili powder, 1 tsp cumin, 1/2 tsp paprika, salt, and pepper.

4. Simmer for 20-25 minutes.

5. Serve topped with 1 tbsp Greek yogurt and 1 tbsp shredded low-fat cheddar cheese.

Day 18

Breakfast: Fruit and nut bar with yogurt

Macronutrients: 350 calories, 20g protein, 45g carbs, 15g fat

Recipe:

1. Choose a high-protein, low-sugar fruit and nut bar (around 200 calories).

2. Serve with 3/4 cup plain Greek yogurt.

3. Top yogurt with 1/4 cup mixed berries.

Lunch: Caprese sandwich

Macronutrients: 400 calories, 20g protein, 40g carbs, 20g fat

Recipe:

1. Take 2 slices of whole grain bread.

2. Layer 2 oz fresh mozzarella cheese, 2 thick slices of tomato, and 5-6 fresh basil leaves.

3. Drizzle with 1 tsp balsamic glaze and 1 tsp olive oil.

4. Season with salt and pepper.

5. Serve with a small side salad of mixed greens and balsamic vinaigrette.

Dinner: Baked tilapia with brown rice

Macronutrients: 420 calories, 35g protein, 45g carbs, 12g fat

Recipe:

1. Preheat oven to 400°F (200°C).

2. Season a 5 oz tilapia fillet with lemon juice, garlic powder, paprika, salt, and pepper.

3. Bake for 12-15 minutes until fish flakes easily with a fork.

4. Cook 1/2 cup brown rice according to package instructions.

5. Steam 1 cup of mixed vegetables (broccoli, carrots, snap peas).

6. Serve fish over rice with vegetables on the side.

Day 19

Breakfast: Breakfast quinoa bowl

Macronutrients: 380 calories, 15g protein, 60g carbs, 12g fat

Recipe:

1. Cook 1/2 cup quinoa in 1 cup water or milk until tender.

2. Stir in 1/2 mashed banana and 1 tsp honey.

3. Top with 1/4 cup mixed berries, 1 tbsp sliced almonds, and a sprinkle of cinnamon.

4. If desired, add a splash of milk before serving.

Lunch: Bean and corn salad

Macronutrients: 350 calories, 15g protein, 55g carbs, 12g fat

Recipe:

1. In a bowl, combine 1/2 cup mixed beans (kidney, black beans), 1/4 cup corn kernels, 1/4 cup diced tomatoes, and 2 tbsp diced red onion.

2. Add 1/4 diced avocado and 2 tbsp chopped cilantro.

3. Dress with 1 tbsp olive oil, 1 tbsp lime juice, salt, and pepper.

4. Serve over 1 cup mixed salad greens.

Dinner: Turkey burger with side salad

Macronutrients: 450 calories, 35g protein, 35g carbs, 20g fat

Recipe:

1. Mix 4 oz ground turkey with 1 tbsp whole wheat breadcrumbs, 1 tsp Dijon mustard, and herbs.

2. Form into a patty and grill or pan-cook until fully cooked.

3. Serve on a whole wheat bun with lettuce, tomato, and 1 tbsp avocado mashed with lemon juice.

4. Pair with a side salad of mixed greens, cucumber, and balsamic vinaigrette.

Day 20

Breakfast: Vegetable juice with boiled eggs

Macronutrients: 300 calories, 18g protein, 30g carbs, 14g fat

Recipe:

1. Prepare 1 cup of low-sodium vegetable juice.

2. Boil 2 eggs for 7 minutes for soft-boiled eggs.

3. Serve eggs with 1 slice whole grain toast and 1 tsp butter.

Lunch: Grilled chicken Caesar salad

Macronutrients: 400 calories, 35g protein, 20g carbs, 22g fat

Recipe:

1. Grill 4 oz chicken breast seasoned with herbs and spices.

2. Chop 2 cups romaine lettuce and toss with 2 tbsp low-fat Caesar dressing.

3. Add sliced grilled chicken, 1 tbsp grated Parmesan cheese, and 5-6 whole grain croutons.

4. Garnish with a lemon wedge.

Dinner: Eggplant parmesan

Macronutrients: 420 calories, 20g protein, 45g carbs, 20g fat

Recipe:

1. Slice 1 small eggplant into 1/2-inch rounds.

2. Dip eggplant slices in beaten egg white, then coat with a mixture of whole wheat breadcrumbs and grated Parmesan.

3. Bake at 400°F (200°C) for 20 minutes, flipping halfway through.

4. Top each slice with 1 tbsp marinara sauce and 1/2 oz low-fat mozzarella.

5. Broil for 2-3 minutes until cheese melts.

6. Serve with 1/2 cup whole wheat pasta tossed with 1 tsp olive oil and herbs.

Day 21

Breakfast: Peanut butter and banana smoothie

Macronutrients: 380 calories, 20g protein, 45g carbs, 18g fat

Recipe:

1. In a blender, combine 1 medium banana, 1 cup unsweetened almond milk, 1 tbsp peanut butter, 1/2 scoop vanilla protein powder, and 1/2 cup ice.

2. Blend until smooth and creamy.

3. If desired, add a sprinkle of cinnamon before serving.

Lunch: Chicken and vegetable soup

Macronutrients: 350 calories, 30g protein, 35g carbs, 10g fat

Recipe:

1. In a pot, sauté 1/4 cup each diced onion, carrot, and celery in 1 tsp olive oil.

2. Add 3 oz diced chicken breast and cook until no longer pink.

3. Add 2 cups low-sodium chicken broth, 1/2 cup diced tomatoes, and 1/2 cup mixed vegetables.

4. Season with herbs, salt, and pepper.

5. Simmer for 20 minutes.

6. Serve with 1 small whole grain roll.

Dinner: Baked salmon with quinoa and broccoli

Macronutrients: 450 calories, 35g protein, 40g carbs, 20g fat

Recipe:

1. Preheat oven to 400°F (200°C).

2. Season a 5 oz salmon fillet with lemon juice, dill, salt, and pepper.

3. Bake for 12-15 minutes until salmon flakes easily.

4. Cook 1/2 cup quinoa according to package instructions.

5. Steam 1 cup broccoli florets.

6. Serve salmon over quinoa with broccoli on the side. Drizzle with 1 tsp olive oil.

Day 22

Breakfast: Whole grain toast with avocado and tomato

Macronutrients: 350 calories, 12g protein, 40g carbs, 20g fat

Recipe:

1. Toast 2 slices of whole grain bread.

2. Mash 1/4 avocado and spread on toast.

3. Top each slice with 2 thin slices of tomato.

4. Sprinkle with salt, pepper, and red pepper flakes if desired.

5. Serve with 1 hard-boiled egg on the side.

Lunch: Quinoa salad with mixed vegetables

Macronutrients: 400 calories, 15g protein, 60g carbs, 16g fat

Recipe:

1. Cook 1/2 cup quinoa according to package instructions and let cool.

2. Mix cooled quinoa with 1 cup mixed chopped vegetables (cucumber, bell peppers, cherry tomatoes).

3. Add 2 tbsp crumbled feta cheese and 1 tbsp chopped fresh herbs (parsley, mint).

4. Dress with 1 tbsp olive oil and 1 tbsp lemon juice.

5. Season with salt and pepper to taste.

Dinner: Chicken fajitas

Macronutrients: 420 calories, 35g protein, 40g carbs, 15g fat

Recipe:

1. Slice 4 oz chicken breast into strips and season with fajita seasoning.

2. In a pan, sauté chicken with 1/2 cup mixed bell peppers and 1/4 cup sliced onions.

3. Warm 2 small whole wheat tortillas.

4. Fill tortillas with chicken and vegetable mixture.

5. Top with 2 tbsp salsa and 1 tbsp plain Greek yogurt.

6. Serve with a side of sliced avocado (about 1/4 of a medium avocado).

Day 23

Breakfast: Veggie and egg white scramble

Macronutrients: 300 calories, 25g protein, 30g carbs, 10g fat

Recipe:

1. In a pan, sauté 1/2 cup mixed vegetables (spinach, mushrooms, bell peppers) in 1 tsp olive oil.

2. Add 3 egg whites and scramble until cooked.

3. Season with salt, pepper, and herbs.

4. Serve with 1 slice whole grain toast and 1 small fruit (like a small apple or orange).

Lunch: Tuna salad on whole grain bread

Macronutrients: 380 calories, 30g protein, 40g carbs, 14g fat

Recipe:

1. Mix 3 oz canned tuna (drained) with 1 tbsp Greek yogurt, 1 tsp Dijon mustard, and 1 tbsp diced celery.

2. Spread on 2 slices of whole grain bread.

3. Add lettuce and tomato slices.

4. Serve with baby carrots and cucumber slices on the side.

Dinner: Lentil and vegetable curry

Macronutrients: 420 calories, 20g protein, 65g carbs, 12g fat

Recipe:

1. In a pot, sauté 1/4 cup diced onion and 1 minced garlic clove in 1 tsp coconut oil.

2. Add 1/2 cup dried red lentils, 1 cup vegetable broth, 1/2 cup coconut milk, and 1 cup mixed vegetables.

3. Season with 1 tbsp curry powder, 1 tsp turmeric, salt, and pepper.

4. Simmer for 20-25 minutes until lentils are tender.

5. Serve over 1/2 cup cooked brown rice and garnish with fresh cilantro.

Day 24

Breakfast: Oatmeal with apple and cinnamon

Macronutrients: 350 calories, 12g protein, 60g carbs, 10g fat

Recipe:

1. Cook 1/2 cup rolled oats with 1 cup water or low-fat milk.

2. Dice 1 small apple and add to the oatmeal during the last minute of cooking.

3. Stir in 1/2 tsp cinnamon and 1 tsp honey.

4. Top with 1 tbsp chopped walnuts.

Lunch: Turkey and hummus wrap

Macronutrients: 400 calories, 25g protein, 45g carbs, 18g fat

Recipe:

1. Spread 2 tbsp hummus on a whole wheat tortilla.

2. Layer 3 oz sliced turkey breast, 1/4 cup mixed greens, 2 slices tomato, and 2 slices cucumber.

3. Roll up tightly and cut in half.

4. Serve with 1 small orange on the side.

Dinner: Grilled sirloin steak with roasted vegetables

Macronutrients: 450 calories, 35g protein, 30g carbs, 22g fat

Recipe:

1. Season a 4 oz sirloin steak with salt and pepper.

2. Grill or pan-sear to desired doneness.

3. Roast 1.5 cups mixed vegetables (Brussels sprouts, carrots, red onion) tossed with 1 tsp olive oil at 400°F (200°C) for 20-25 minutes.

4. Serve steak with roasted vegetables and 1/2 small baked sweet potato.

Day 25

Breakfast: Peanut butter banana toast

Macronutrients: 380 calories, 15g protein, 50g carbs, 18g fat

Recipe:

1. Toast 2 slices of whole grain bread.

2. Spread 1 tbsp peanut butter on each slice.

3. Top with 1 sliced banana.

4. Sprinkle with chia seeds and a drizzle of honey if desired.

Lunch: Veggie burger with side salad

Macronutrients: 400 calories, 20g protein, 45g carbs, 18g fat

Recipe:

1. Cook a store-bought veggie burger according to package instructions.

2. Serve on a whole wheat bun with lettuce, tomato, and 1 tbsp guacamole.

3. Pair with a side salad of mixed greens, cucumber, and 1 tbsp light vinaigrette.

Dinner: Baked cod with quinoa and broccoli

Macronutrients: 420 calories, 35g protein, 45g carbs, 10g fat

Recipe:

1. Preheat oven to 400°F (200°C).

2. Season a 5 oz cod fillet with lemon juice, garlic, and herbs.

3. Bake for 12-15 minutes until fish flakes easily.

4. Cook 1/2 cup quinoa according to package instructions.

5. Steam 1 cup broccoli florets.

6. Serve cod over quinoa with broccoli on the side.

Day 26

Breakfast: Green smoothie

Macronutrients: 300 calories, 20g protein, 45g carbs, 8g fat

Recipe:

1. In a blender, combine 1 cup spinach, 1/2 banana, 1/2 cup frozen mango, 1 scoop vanilla protein powder, 1 cup unsweetened almond milk, and 1/2 cup ice.

2. Blend until smooth and creamy.

Lunch: Grilled chicken and avocado salad

Macronutrients: 420 calories, 35g protein, 20g carbs, 25g fat

Recipe:

1. Grill 4 oz chicken breast seasoned with herbs and spices.

2. Prepare a salad with 2 cups mixed greens, 1/4 avocado (diced), 1/4 cup cherry tomatoes, and 2 tbsp sliced almonds.

3. Dress with 1 tbsp olive oil and 1 tbsp balsamic vinegar.

4. Top salad with sliced grilled chicken.

Dinner: Vegetarian stir-fry with tofu

Macronutrients: 400 calories, 25g protein, 50g carbs, 15g fat

Recipe:

1. Press and cube 4 oz firm tofu.

2. Stir-fry tofu in 1 tsp sesame oil until golden.

3. Add 1.5 cups mixed vegetables (bell peppers, broccoli, carrots, snap peas) and stir-fry until tender-crisp.

4. Add 1 tbsp low-sodium soy sauce and 1 tsp honey.

5. Serve over 1/2 cup cooked brown rice.

Day 27

Breakfast: Whole grain English muffin with nut butter

Macronutrients: 350 calories, 15g protein, 40g carbs, 18g fat

Recipe:

1. Toast 1 whole grain English muffin.

2. Spread 1 tbsp almond or peanut butter on each half.

3. Top with 1/2 sliced banana and a sprinkle of cinnamon.

4. Serve with 1 small orange on the side.

Lunch: Vegetable and bean soup

Macronutrients: 380 calories, 18g protein, 60g carbs, 10g fat

Recipe:

1. In a pot, sauté 1/4 cup each diced onion, carrot, and celery in 1 tsp olive oil.

2. Add 1/2 cup mixed beans, 2 cups vegetable broth, 1/2 cup diced tomatoes, and 1 cup chopped mixed vegetables.

3. Season with herbs, salt, and pepper.

4. Simmer for 20-25 minutes.

5. Serve with 1 small whole grain roll.

Dinner: Lean beef kabobs with vegetables

Macronutrients: 420 calories, 35g protein, 30g carbs, 18g fat

Recipe:

1. Cut 4 oz lean beef into cubes and marinate in 1 tbsp olive oil, lemon juice, and herbs.

2. Thread beef and 1 cup mixed vegetables (bell peppers, onions, zucchini) onto skewers.

3. Grill or broil for 10-12 minutes, turning occasionally.

4. Serve with 1/2 cup cooked quinoa and a side of tzatziki sauce (2 tbsp Greek yogurt mixed with cucumber and dill).

Day 28

Breakfast: Greek yogurt parfait

Macronutrients: 350 calories, 25g protein, 45g carbs, 10g fat

Recipe:

1. Layer 1 cup plain Greek yogurt with 1/4 cup low-fat granola and 1/2 cup mixed berries.

2. Drizzle with 1 tsp honey if desired.

Lunch: Turkey and cheese roll-ups with fruit

Macronutrients: 400 calories, 30g protein, 35g carbs, 20g fat

Recipe:

1. Roll 3 oz sliced turkey breast with 1 oz low-fat cheese and 1/4 sliced avocado.

2. Secure with toothpicks if needed.

3. Serve with 1 cup mixed raw vegetables (carrots, cucumber, bell peppers) and 1 small apple.

Dinner: Grilled chicken with zucchini noodles

Macronutrients: 420 calories, 40g protein, 25g carbs, 18g fat

Recipe:

1. Grill 5 oz chicken breast seasoned with herbs and spices.

2. Spiralize 2 medium zucchinis into noodles.

3. Sauté zucchini noodles in 1 tsp olive oil with 1 minced garlic clove.

4. Toss zucchini noodles with 2 tbsp marinara sauce and 1 tbsp grated Parmesan cheese.

5. Serve sliced grilled chicken over zucchini noodles.

Day 29

Breakfast: Vegetable omelet

Macronutrients: 350 calories, 25g protein, 20g carbs, 22g fat

Recipe:

1. Whisk 2 whole eggs and 1 egg white with salt and pepper.

2. Sauté 1/2 cup mixed vegetables (spinach, mushrooms, bell peppers) in 1 tsp olive oil.

3. Pour eggs over vegetables and cook until set.

4. Fold omelet and top with 1 tbsp crumbled feta cheese.

5. Serve with 1 slice whole grain toast.

Lunch: Mediterranean quinoa bowl

Macronutrients: 420 calories, 18g protein, 55g carbs, 20g fat

Recipe:

1. Cook 1/2 cup quinoa according to package instructions.

2. Mix cooled quinoa with 1/4 cup diced cucumber, 1/4 cup halved cherry tomatoes, 2 tbsp diced red onion, and 5 sliced kalamata olives.

3. Add 2 oz crumbled feta cheese and 1 tbsp chopped fresh parsley.

4. Dress with 1 tbsp olive oil and 1 tbsp lemon juice.

Dinner: Baked eggplant with tomato sauce

Macronutrients: 380 calories, 15g protein, 45g carbs, 18g fat

Recipe:

1. Slice 1 small eggplant and brush with 1 tsp olive oil.

2. Bake eggplant slices at 400°F (200°C) for 20 minutes, flipping halfway through.

3. Top each slice with 2 tbsp marinara sauce and 1 tbsp part-skim mozzarella cheese.

4. Broil for 2-3 minutes until cheese melts.

5. Serve with 1/2 cup whole wheat pasta tossed with 1 tsp olive oil and fresh basil.

Day 30

Breakfast: Whole grain cereal with berries and milk

Macronutrients: 350 calories, 15g protein, 60g carbs, 8g fat

Recipe:

1. Pour 1 cup whole grain, high-fiber cereal into a bowl.

2. Add 1 cup low-fat milk or unsweetened plant-based milk.

3. Top with 1/2 cup mixed berries and 1 tbsp chopped nuts.

Lunch: Egg salad on whole grain bread

Macronutrients: 400 calories, 25g protein, 35g carbs, 20g fat

Recipe:

1. Mash 2 hard-boiled eggs with 1 tbsp Greek yogurt, 1 tsp Dijon mustard, and 1 tbsp diced celery.

2. Spread on 2 slices of whole grain bread.

3. Add lettuce and tomato slices.

4. Serve with carrot sticks and cucumber slices on the side.

Dinner: Baked salmon with roasted vegetables

Macronutrients: 450 calories, 35g protein, 30g carbs, 22g fat

Recipe:

1. Preheat oven to 400°F (200°C).

2. Season a 5 oz salmon fillet with lemon juice, dill, salt, and pepper.

3. Roast 1.5 cups mixed vegetables (Brussels sprouts, sweet potato cubes, red onion) tossed with 1 tsp olive oil.

4. Bake salmon and vegetables for 12-15 minutes until salmon flakes easily and vegetables are tender.

5. Serve with 1/4 cup cooked quinoa.

Remember to stay hydrated by drinking plenty of water throughout the day, and adjust portion sizes as needed based on individual caloric needs and activity levels. It's also important to consult with a healthcare professional or registered dietitian before starting any new diet plan.

Grocery Shopping List for the 30 Day Meal Plan by Week

Week 1 (Days 1-7) Grocery List

Produce:

- Mixed berries (strawberries, blueberries, raspberries)

- Bananas

- Lemons

- Mixed salad greens

- Spinach

- Cucumbers

- Tomatoes

- Bell peppers (various colors)

- Onions

- Garlic

- Carrots

- Broccoli

- Zucchini

- Green beans

- Asparagus

- Avocados

Proteins:

- Chicken breasts

- Salmon fillets

- Lean ground turkey

- Eggs

- Tofu (firm)

- Canned tuna

Dairy and Alternatives:

- Greek yogurt

- Low-fat milk or unsweetened plant-based milk

- Feta cheese

- Low-fat mozzarella cheese

- Parmesan cheese

Grains and Legumes:

- Rolled oats

- Quinoa

- Brown rice

- Whole grain bread

- Whole wheat tortillas

- Whole wheat pasta

- Canned black beans

- Canned kidney beans

- Lentils

Nuts and Seeds:

- Almonds

- Chia seeds

Other:

- Olive oil

- Balsamic vinegar

- Low-sodium vegetable broth

- Low-sodium chicken broth

- Marinara sauce

- Hummus

- Dijon mustard

- Low-fat granola

Week 2 (Days 8-14) Grocery List

Produce:

- Mixed berries

- Bananas

- Lemons

- Mixed salad greens

- Spinach

- Romaine lettuce

- Cucumbers

- Tomatoes

- Cherry tomatoes

- Bell peppers

- Onions

- Garlic

- Carrots

- Broccoli

- Zucchini

- Eggplant

- Green beans

- Mushrooms

- Celery

- Fresh herbs (basil, cilantro, parsley)

Proteins:

- Chicken breasts

- Salmon fillets

- Lean ground turkey

- Eggs

- Shrimp

- Canned tuna

- Lean sirloin steak

Dairy and Alternatives:

- Greek yogurt

- Low-fat milk or unsweetened plant-based milk

- Feta cheese

- Low-fat mozzarella cheese

- Parmesan cheese

- Cottage cheese

Grains and Legumes:

- Quinoa

- Brown rice

- Whole grain bread

- Whole wheat buns

- Whole wheat pasta

- Canned chickpeas

Nuts and Seeds:

- Almonds

- Walnuts

Other:

- Olive oil

- Balsamic vinegar

- Low-sodium soy sauce

- Sesame oil

- Low-sodium vegetable broth

- Marinara sauce

- Dijon mustard

- Peanut butter or almond butter

Week 3 (Days 15-21) Grocery List

Produce:

- Mixed berries

- Bananas

- Lemons

- Apples

- Oranges

- Mixed salad greens

- Spinach

- Cucumbers

- Tomatoes

- Cherry tomatoes

- Bell peppers

- Onions

- Garlic

- Carrots

- Broccoli

- Zucchini

- Sweet potatoes

- Green beans

- Mushrooms

- Celery

- Fresh herbs (basil, cilantro, parsley, mint)

Proteins:

- Chicken breasts

- Salmon fillets

- Lean ground turkey

- Eggs

- Tofu (firm)

- Canned tuna

- Lean pork tenderloin

Dairy and Alternatives:

- Greek yogurt

- Low-fat milk or unsweetened plant-based milk

- Feta cheese

- Low-fat mozzarella cheese

- Parmesan cheese

Grains and Legumes:

- Rolled oats

- Quinoa

- Brown rice

- Whole grain bread

- Whole wheat tortillas

- Whole wheat pasta

- Canned black beans

- Lentils

Nuts and Seeds:

- Almonds

- Chia seeds

Other:

- Olive oil

- Balsamic vinegar

- Coconut milk

- Low-sodium vegetable broth

- Low-sodium chicken broth

- Marinara sauce

- Hummus

- Dijon mustard

- Peanut butter or almond butter

- Protein powder (vanilla)

Week 4 (Days 22-30) Grocery List

Produce:

- Mixed berries

- Bananas

- Lemons

- Apples

- Oranges

- Mixed salad greens

- Spinach

- Cucumbers

- Tomatoes

- Cherry tomatoes

- Bell peppers

- Onions

- Garlic

- Carrots

- Broccoli

- Zucchini

- Sweet potatoes

- Green beans

- Mushrooms

- Brussels sprouts

- Eggplant

- Fresh herbs (basil, cilantro, parsley, dill)

Proteins:

- Chicken breasts

- Salmon fillets

- Lean ground beef

- Eggs

- Tofu (firm)

- Canned tuna

- Lean sirloin steak

- Cod fillets

Dairy and Alternatives:

- Greek yogurt

- Low-fat milk or unsweetened plant-based milk

- Feta cheese

- Low-fat mozzarella cheese

- Parmesan cheese

Grains and Legumes:

- Quinoa

- Brown rice

- Whole grain bread

- Whole grain English muffins

- Whole wheat pasta

- Canned mixed beans

- High-fiber whole grain cereal

Nuts and Seeds:

- Almonds

- Mixed nuts

Other:

- Olive oil

- Balsamic vinegar

- Low-sodium vegetable broth

- Marinara sauce

- Dijon mustard

- Peanut butter or almond butter

- Whole grain crackers

Remember to adjust quantities based on your personal needs and preferences. Also, check your pantry before shopping to avoid buying items you already have on hand.